Women's Natural Guidebook

8 Simple and Natural Steps to Enjoy Holistic Fitness and Greatness!

Dr. Lynn Migdal

Doctor of Chiropractic and ChiroChi Master

Disclaimer: The purpose of this guidebook is to educate and to entertain. The author and publisher do not guarantee that anyone following these ideas, suggestions, tips or strategies will be successful. The author and publisher shall have neither liability nor responsibility to anyone with respect to any loss, or damage allegedly caused, directly or indirectly, by the information in this book. This guidebook is not a substitute for the advice of a physician. The reader should always consult a physician in matters of his/her health, especially with any symptoms that might require diagnosis or medical attention.

ISBN-13: 978-0-61599-211-2

Migdal Chiropractic and Family Wellness Center
Phone: 561-278-2224 • Fax: 561-278-2399
lookingupthemovement.com • ChiroChi.com

Dr. Lynn Migdal, wellness Chiropractor, author, inspirational speaker, and holistic fitness expert, dedicates this book to all the women in the world who are suffering in their bodies and in their lives. Her dream is for all women, young and old, to empower themselves and increase their potential for health and happiness.

I wish to thank my mother, my sister, my daughters, and my friends Jeorgie and Eleanor for all their loving lessons and gifts. I appreciate the rough times, the joyous times and the magnificent journey we have traveled together!

Contents

About Dr. Lynn Ann Migdal, vii

The 8 Healing Steps to Greatness, 1

STEP 1

Honor Your Powerful, Feminine, Innate Ability for Health and Greatness, 3

STEP 2

Become Neurologically Fit at Any Age, 5

STEP 3

Choose Emotion Fitness: The Road to Healthy Cycles and Female Greatness!, 9

STEP 4

Balance Your Pelvis and Untip Your Uterus, 26

STEP 5

Practice Spinal Hygiene All Day Long, 29

STEP 6

Reduce Toxic Thoughts and Foods That Can Cause Hormonal Imbalances, 35

STEP 7

Choose Holistic Feminine Fitness and Enjoy Total Health, 42

STEP 8

Embrace the ChiroChi® Lifestyle All Day Long, 46

Other Natural Holistic Healing Books by Dr. Lynn Ann Migdal, 51

About Dr. Lynn Ann Migdal

Dr. Migdal graduated from the New York School of Chiropractic in 1981. Her fresh outlook on disease prevention, holistic neurological fitness and spinal hygiene has helped thousands of people, young and old, to live up to their highest physical and mental potential. In the past 30 years she has owned and directed three successful Natural Healing Centers in Delray Beach, Florida. She is highly regarded by her peers and patients for her holistic views on fitness and health.

The programs Dr. Migdal offers are educational, exciting and fun. They are packed with information on health and wellness that all people can enjoy. She teaches about the body's natural ability to heal itself which, when combined with her Wellness and Fitness Programs, allow people to achieve success in all areas of life. As a result, many of her students and patients have weaned themselves off potentially harm- ful drugs. Others have found surgical procedures unnecessary due to the benefits they received under her expert guidance.

Dr. Migdal is the author of Wind Kissed, a self-empowering fantasy novel for children and parents. She has also written Student's Natural Guide to Greatness, a simple guidebook to teach students of all ages how to increase their levels of total fitness, success and health, and Sacred Birth Promise an autobiography.

In addition to her writing accomplishments, Dr. Migdal is also an expert in the field of Family Wellness. She is a Family Wellness Chiropractor, a Reiki and ChiroChi™ Master, an Energy Intuitive, a Holistic Healer, and is a Dancing Breath of Life Wellness Coach. She is a great source of healing to all those she touches with her knowledge, her inspiring lectures and numerous holistic programs. Dr. Migdal encourages people to take the "holistic approach" to life and healing so that they experience the great benefits of peace and total wellness.

"Learning easy, natural, chemical, emotional, and physical stress solutions enhances any woman's ability to succeed. A woman's success is in direct proportion to her internal state of wellness; increasing her level of wellness will always increase her level of success!"

—Dr. Lynn Ann Migdal

The 8 Healing Steps
to Greatness

1. Honor Your Powerful, Feminine, Innate Ability for Health and Greatness

2. Become Neurologically Fit at Any Age

3. Choose Emotional Fitness: the Road to Healthy Cycles and Female Greatness

4. Balance Your Pelvis and Untip Your Uterus

5. Practice Spinal Hygiene All Day Long

6. Reduce Toxic Thoughts and Foods That Create Hormonal Imbalance

7. Increase Holistic Feminine Fitness and Enjoy Total Health

8. Embrace the ChiroChi™ Lifestyle

Honor Your Powerful, Feminine, Innate Ability for Health and Greatness

*Females Are Powerful and Are Born
for Health and Greatness!*

All women are born for greatness! You are a miraculous, creative spirit who was born to be happy, healthy, and terrific! You are powerful, and you have the ability to create life, carry life and to deliver life. The creative magical powers that you were born with are living inside of you and are waiting to be nourished and honored.

Women are special and very powerful beings! Most of you do not understand how very special you really are. Women's natural healing powers have been stolen from them, and it is my mission to re-educate women to empower themselves. You see, all women are born with the ability to naturally heal themselves and to express greatness. All have a smart doctor living inside of them who knows how to heal. In this book I'll refer to this doctor as the "Innate Intelligence." Your miraculous innate intelligence runs the functioning of every cell, system and organ in your body.

As a 59-year-old woman, I've experienced most of the unhealthy symptoms from which women endure. I have had premenstrual and menstrual blues, pain, and suffered from painful menstrual cramps, anger and headaches. I've experienced pregnancy with its nausea, dizziness, headaches, numbness and back pain. I've gone through the miraculous and blissful delivery of my two beautiful daughters. I have successfully experienced the balancing act of breastfeeding my babies and being a busy doctor. I've also gone through menopause with very little discomfort. All the information in this book comes from my personal experience as a woman, as well as my 32 years as a wellness Chiropractor and holistic healer.

I have experienced the joy of being naturally healed through Chiropractic care! My pre- and postmenstrual problems and my menstrual cramps were taken away early in Chiropractic school with specific spinal and pelvic adjustments. My morning sickness was healed in two Chiropractic visits early in my pregnancy. My pregnancy symptoms of lower back pain, leg pains, ankle swelling, dizziness, headaches and numbness were also taken away by Chiropractic in a couple of visits. Two years before I became pregnant, I was paralyzed from an allergic reaction to a vaccine. I feared that I would not be strong enough to go through labor. I am proud to say that even a weak female can go through a safe and natural labor and delivery. I have also experienced help by Chiropractic adjustments when I was having a problem breast feeding. Chiropractic adjustments have relieved me of hot flashes and allowed me to go through menopause gracefully without any supplemental hormones.

I am thankful to Chiropractic and its natural ability to balance my female body and assist my own natural healing powers.

I have had the privilege of helping thousands of women heal and balance their female cycles. Inside every woman there is an innate intelligence that knows how to create health and wellness. Women need to understand their anatomy and learn how to take control of their health. When women want to choose natural methods of healing, they must realize that it is an inside job. When women realize their greatness and take control of their own health they become more powerful and happy.

From one cell to two cells, from two cells to four cells, all of us grew our organs and all of our systems after we were conceived. That miracle of life that you performed in your mother's womb is still inside you. We women are amazing creatures! No matter how old you are, you are still a miraculous, marvelous part of this great, creative universe. If you are suffering and having difficulty believing me, just prick your finger and watch your skin grow back from inside out. Remember, from now on all healing comes from within you!

You are an intelligent, powerful being who has the power to naturally heal herself and create an abundant life of joy, health, and peace!

I'd like you to get some "mental dental floss," and place it in one ear. Imagine pulling it through your skull out the other ear, removing all negative thoughts and beliefs you're holding onto that are limiting and unhealthy. Use this mental dental floss whenever you're having doubts that you are very powerful and full of miracles.

STEP 2

Become Neurologically Fit
at Any Age

A woman's brain and nervous system control the functioning of her entire body. So no matter what age or state of health she is in, when she learns how to increase her level of neurological fitness, she improves the state of her health. Not one part of the body functions on its own without direct communication from the nervous system.

What is neurological fitness you ask? It is the state in which your nervous system functions at 100%. It is the healthy physical, chemical, emotional and mental balance of the nervous system which allows it and the rest of the body to function at its optimum. When a woman learns and practices neurological fitness, she becomes holistically fit and enhances the vital energy from her brain to her body.

The bones of the cranium, spine and pelvis were created to hold this very important nervous system in place and to protect it from harm. There is a direct relationship between the health and alignment of these bones and the ability of the nervous system to be healthy and fit. Chiropractic is a natural, holistic approach to neurological fitness and health. When Chiropractic releases pressure off of the nervous system, it creates a holistic healthy shift physically, chemically, emotionally and spiritually. This reduces stress on all levels and promotes health and wellness.

To understand neurological fitness, use the Autonomic Nervous System chart at the end of this chapter to trace the nerves as they exit the spine and go to the organs. Remember that Chiropractors are holistic and, although the chart shows the specific areas where specific nerves exit the spine and their direct pathways to the organs, a Chiropractor may need to adjust other levels of the spine below or above these areas to assist the nerves to these organs as well. Chiropractic removes pressure and energy blockages from the entire nervous system. Often lower areas in the spine that are out of place can cause higher areas of the spine to move out of place. The opposite is true as well: the main cause of dysfunction to lower areas can be from higher areas of the spine. Think of the spinal column as a rope or string. When you twist the top the rest of the rope follows and twists. So stay open to a holistic approach to the empowerment of your whole nervous system.

The autonomic nervous system functions automatically, and most of the time it is taken for granted. If a healthy reproductive system is your goal, then you must increase the neurological fitness of your lower back as these nerves control the function of that system. Pressure on the lower back can also have a negative effect on the cranial bones and the pituitary gland. The nervous system at this level of the spine also controls your lower limbs, kidneys, urinary system, adrenals, and bowels to function. Remember that the pressure in your lower back may be coming from your upper back or neck.

You can see by the chart that to have a healthy digestive system you need to have a healthy state of neurological fitness in your middle back area. The nerves to the liver come out of the middle of your back (thoracic area) and help control your cholesterol and your ability to detoxify poisons. The nerves to the pancreas, also emanating out of this area, control your insulin levels. The nerves to your stomach control the levels of stomach acids and enzymes. Becoming conscious of your posture in your middle back can also affect the nerves to the spleen, which are involved with red blood cells and your immune system.

If you want a healthier circulatory system or respiratory system, you need to assist the nerves in your upper back to be happy, fit and free of pressure. Many women who keep their shoulders and upper back area rounded, hunched, or twisted for long periods of time have problems with their breathing and/or with their blood pressure.

The nerves going through the neck are responsible for the functioning of most of your body, **including the aforementioned areas**. The neck is the closest to the brain and brainstem and, therefore, is the most important part of the spine. The nerves of the neck also go directly to the face and control your eyes, ears, nose, teeth, throat, upper limbs and sinus area. If you want any part of your body to be healthy, take care of the nerves that go through your neck.

The brain is in charge of the entire nervous system and controls the functioning of all your cells, systems and organs. Increasing the neurological fitness of your cranial nerves and your brain will improve your total health, and your ability to heal yourself of disease. Becoming more conscious of your possible one-sided jaw clenching, and reducing your head tilt will help your cranial bones and your brain function.

The most important thing to remember here is that your state of health is in direct proportion to your level of neurological fitness.

No matter what your diagnosis or prognosis, no matter what medicine or surgery you have experienced, and no matter how old you are, increased health and fitness of your nervous system can give you more vital energy and make you healthier. Please remember that the nervous system is a system of communication. Improving neurological fitness increases the flow of communication from the brain to the body. Since the nervous system runs all the other systems, it needs the most care.

One of the most important things that is usually overlooked in health care is that the nervous system controls the immune system. To increase natural immunity you must take the time to create neurological fitness. Chiropractors are natural neurologists who care for the nervous system using natural means. Gentle, specific Chiropractic adjustments remove nerve interference that can be caused by vertebrae and other bones that are out of alignment. You cannot achieve neurological fitness if you are living with unhappy, unhealthy, pressured nerves to your organs.

Most Chiropractic patients are able to reduce, or completely get off, the toxic yeast- producing effect of the overuse of antibiotics. Millions of people are choosing Chiropractic care to empower their immune systems and are successfully raising their natural levels of immunity.

Your level of natural immunity is in direct proportion to your level of neurological fitness.

As a woman experiencing the miracles of her body's natural ability to heal itself from female problems and as a doctor watching thousands of women heal naturally, I can assure you that you were born to heal yourself. The wonders of the human body and its miraculous ability to create life and health are inside of you waiting to be experienced. Treat your nervous system well because when it is happy and strong your body is healthy and strong!

The nervous system is very sensitive to stress. To be healthy, women must learn to reduce stress on all levels. The foods a woman eats, the thoughts she thinks, the emotions she feels, and her posture all determine her level of neurological fitness.

Unfortunately, we are a symptomatic-based medical society where many believe if they are not experiencing any discomfort, that they are healthy. The definition of health is when the body is functioning at 100% and not just the absence of symptoms or disease.

To be really healthy and in great condition, become conscious of your spinal column and nervous system every day, all day long, and not just when you are sick or in pain.

Most people think you have to have pain to see a Chiropractor. This isn't true. Chiropractors are also preventative, holistic, wellness doctors. They keep women in top neurological fitness and help prevent disease. Many parts of our body do not have pain receptors, so one can be experiencing less nerve flow to an organ and never know it.

A prime example is when a woman's arteries are clogged and she has no clue until five years later when she has chest pain and the doctor tells her she needs open heart surgery. Why didn't she know her heart was not functioning at 100% during those years? If she had experienced chest pain, pain down her arm, jaw pain, or pain in her neck earlier, she might have checked her heart, but because she had no pain or no other symptoms, she presumed she was healthy and didn't go to the doctor until she had pain and it was too late. The lesson here is don't wait for pain to be conscious of your spinal and neurological health.

Another great example is when women have cervical or breast cancer and are not experiencing any symptoms. Unfortunately, after living with cancer for years and not knowing it, they wake up one day in pain, or go for their yearly check-up—and they learn they've had cancer for years.

If you only rely on pain or other symptoms, you can miss the fact that your spine and nervous system might be sick and unable to take great care of your organs. This can go on for many years before you know that you are in a diseased state. We can have clogged arteries or cancer and not have any symptoms.

Daily self-care of your spine and nervous system, and regular preventative check-ups by a Chiropractor, (natural neurologist) can keep your nervous system in tip-top shape.

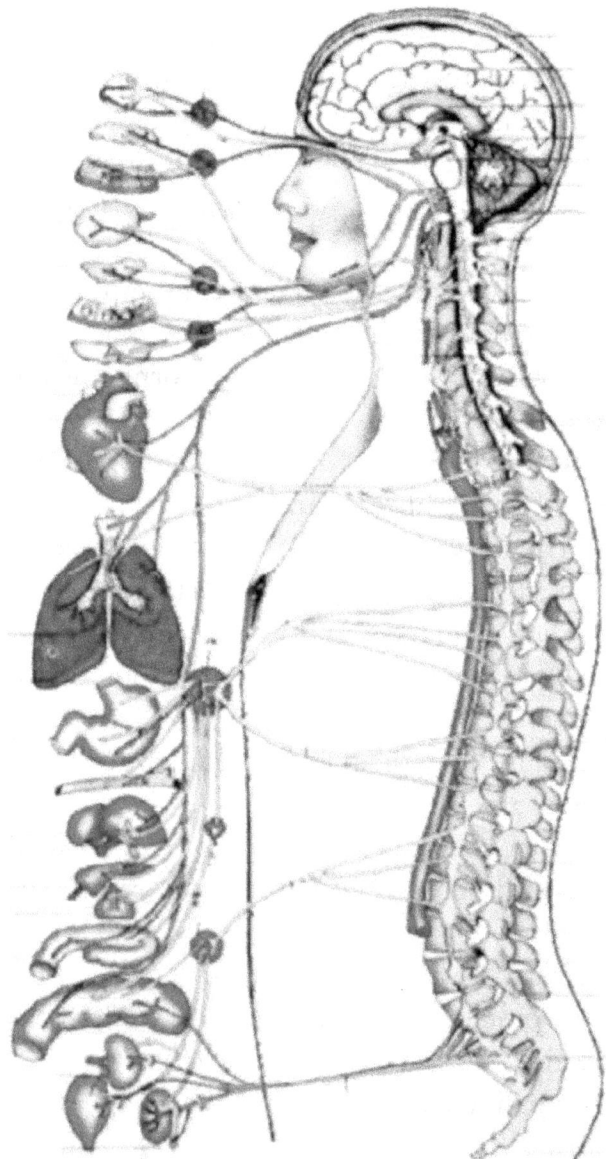

Autonomic
Nervous System

Choose Emotion Fitness:
The Road to Healthy Cycles
and Female Greatness!

Choose is the most important word in this step. You choose your thoughts and you choose to experience the emotions you allow yourself to feel. We've all heard that stress can kill us. Women need to realize they must reduce stress if they want to be healthy. Emotional stress is one way female cycles and hormones can get out of balance.

The interaction between mind and body was proven in cancer research over 30 years ago. Doctors and scientists now know that love and laughter stimulate the immune system's ability to flush cancer cells out of the body. They also know the emotions of anger and resentment negatively affect healing. Interferon is a chemical that is produced by the body to increase the immune system's natural ability to fight disease and to release cancer cells. Its levels go up and down with these emotions. There you have it! Your emotions have chemical reactions that either heal or hurt you. It's not just a theory or belief; it's a fact of life.

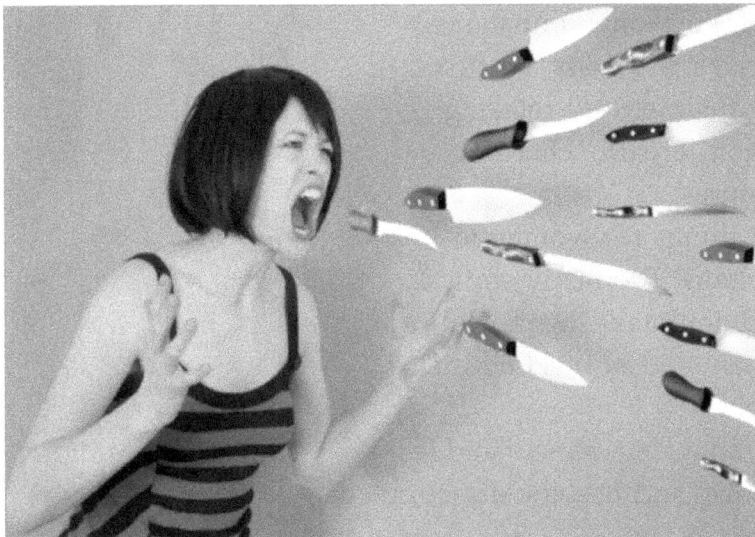

What negative emotions or thoughts are stuck in your heart and mind that you need to let go of? What could you possibly change, release and heal that is keeping you from enjoying your female cycles and health in the rest of your body?

Toxic thoughts and feelings can be more dangerous to women than toxic foods. A healthy diet creates healthy hormonal balance. Thoughts and emotions can affect the digestion of food. The stress of unhealed emotions and constant negative thinking can cause the healthiest of diets to backfire and produce hormonal imbalance and stress in the female organs.

When we're thinking negative thoughts and feeling negative emotions, we might be holding our breath and clenching our buttocks and/or jaw muscles. This can cause stress in the pituitary gland and may tip the uterus. The pituitary runs most of our hormones, so we need to keep it balanced and happy. When we clench our temporal-mandible joint (TMJ) unevenly, it can slightly twist our cranial bones to that side and possibly cause an irregular tug on the pituitary. If the pituitary gland is unhappy or under stress, most of our hormones will not function properly. So when you are stressed, relax your jaw, relax your buttock muscles, and take extra breaths.

Clenching your jaw can also cause cranial pressure that can upset the functioning of your salivary glands and nerves. Being conscious of your jaw and your breath helps your saliva nerves to create the right ph for digestion. Relaxing before, during, and after eating allows your digestion to improve and helps you to balance your hormones.

When you feel stressed out, take a breath and think about your buttock muscles. Are you holding an emotional "butt fist" on one side? Are you sitting and tensely holding your thighs and legs crossed, clenching your pelvic muscles unevenly and causing your pelvis and uterus to twist? Women are given medicine to relieve their symptoms of hormonal imbalance while many can heal themselves naturally by just becoming more conscious of their stress, relaxing their muscles, monitoring their breath, choosing healthy foods and healthy postures.

One of the most important things for women to learn is **not** to ignore their feelings. Too many stuff or push their feelings aside and don't take the time to feel their emotions. Stuffing them and not feeling them is worse than experiencing them.

Anger, guilt, sadness, frustration, resentment and fear are all low-energy negative emotions, and become disastrous if we don't allow them to surface.

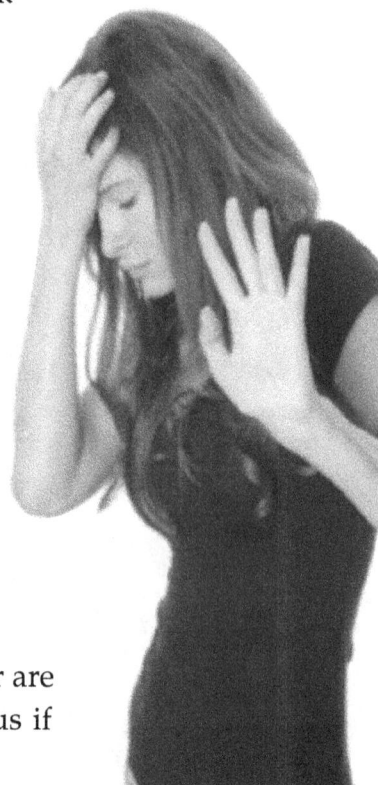

Feeling one's feelings and releasing them in a healthy way can balance a woman's body, mind and spirit. Unfortunately, we live in a society that encourages medicating away our feelings. Women who cry a lot and naturally express their feelings are given drugs to stop crying and to prevent them from feeling sad. Women who have anxiety are given drugs to suppress their fears and never learn to face or release them. These drugs are toxic to our livers, harm our nervous systems, and can cause hormonal problems and female diseases.

After you feel your feelings, it's important to choose peace. Emotional fitness occurs when you live your life surrendering, accepting and being thankful in the NOW!

Are you in the present most of the time? Or are you dwelling on the bad things that happened in your past? Are you constantly in the future, fearful of the bad things that could possibly happen in the next hour, tomorrow, next week or next year? How much of your day is focusing on the negative past or scary future? Are you spending time feeling guilty when you choose your own needs over the needs of others?

We are the only thinkers of our thoughts. Yes, I said to honor your feelings and to release them in a healthy way. I'm not saying to pretend the past was great and that nothing bad can happen in your future. **I'm saying we have the ability to choose peace at any time.** Whenever we want, we can bring our thoughts back to the present time where we are safe. It's healing to think of the past when we concentrate on what was good and happy. It's also healthy to realize what gifts and lessons the negative past has given us. While it can be harmful to the nervous system to spend time worrying about the future, it's very healing to dream about the future and visualize what you'd like to create in your body and in your life.

Many women claim they cannot stop worrying about their family or someone they love. They grew up thinking worry equals love. Women also say they can't stop feeling guilty about the past. They grew up learning from their parents that guilt was attached to love.

Love is the opposite of fear, worry and guilt!

The glorious peace of mind that comes from accepting and surrendering to what is taking place in the present, can help a woman to balance her hormones and create health in her life!

Twelve Step programs teach people to take one day at a time. During a whole day, thousands of negative thoughts of the past or future can fly by without being realized or corrected. Hours and days filled with resentment and/or worry, can waste your precious life, upset your immune system and restrict the natural flow of your cycles. Being conscious of your thoughts, one thought at a time, can help you to stay in the present and cut down on the time you might be dwelling on the negative past or future.

If you cannot surrender and accept your present situation, think about what you are thankful for. Gratitude can bring the mind to a peaceful and happy present. Some women cannot think of anything to be thankful for. To them I say, be thankful for your breath or for the sky. Go outside and breathe and be thankful for whomever and whatever you see. Choosing an attitude of gratitude will help heal your body, mind and spirit.

Both conscious and unconscious unhealed memories of past emotional, physical or sexual abuse can create pain in the pelvis, cause stress, and produce disease. Unforgiving cells full of anger and resentment can keep an abused woman struggling to be healthy and happy. If you were abused in the past, it's important that you see a specialist who deals with anger release. You must feel your true feelings before you can experience true healing. Once anger is truly acknowledged and expressed, a woman can forgive her abusers. This sounds impossible to many women who have experienced abuse. If women hold anger in and never truly forgive, they can create hormonal imbalances and possibly hold cancerous cells in the organs near the abused area.

Forgive all of your abusers and let go of your past for holistic fitness. Forgiveness is done to heal yourself. I was sexually abused on my diaper table and again when I was eighteen. I was also emotionally abused until I was 27. I know the pain and fear abused women feel. I also know the joy of letting it all go, and releasing and forgiving my abusers. When one can joyously release and forgive the past, one can easily cleanse oneself of the manifestation of these thoughts and emotions and unwanted cells in the body. This is not an easy path. Most like to stay in the victim role and never move on to the flow of forgiveness and healing. Many women just medicate their symptoms away and remain unconscious of the true cause of why they are ill.

I thank Chiropractic for helping me to heal all of my female problems and diseases, and I'm also thankful I had the courage to release the emotions that were causing these problems. Healing the past releases toxins from the cells and makes room for the fresh and healthy cells to flourish.

Remember that forgiveness without releasing anger isn't true forgiveness and may not have great results.

Being born the "wrong" sex can cause a woman to feel that she is not wanted and never good enough. In the past, it was often thought it was better if a son were born first. Many women who are first born may have known in the womb that they were supposed to be a boy and were born feeling not good enough. This can also happen when the second and third siblings are the same sex as the first! This "not good enough syndrome" may manifest as a female disease. The syndrome of never feeling

12

good enough as a woman may cause unhealthy stress on the nervous system. Many women feel they are not good enough as a mother, not good enough as a daughter, sister or lover. These issues cause many women to become super women and over-achievers who thrive on stress. They're always looking for approval and appreciation and are often frustrated and depressed when they don't receive them. They judge themselves too strongly and believe they are not good enough as women. Many unconsciously recreate patterns that prove they are not good enough! Learning about one's birth and childhood patterns, and forgiving parents and siblings, can stop the pains of the past. Women are powerful and smart enough to create new patterns of health and happiness.

There are women who stay in unhealthy relationships because they are afraid to leave. They sleep with, live with, and have sex with men they do not respect or love. This is called the "prostitute syndrome" (from The Wisdom of Menopause by Christiane Northrup, M.D., Bantum: New York, 2006) and can cause terrible problems in women's bodies. One problem can be terrible pain in the groin that medicine cannot help. Another is insomnia that occurs when women continue to sleep with men whom they really want to leave. They can toss and turn with night sweats and wake up exhausted. Night sweats, like most female symptoms, have a physical, mental, chemical and emotional cause.

Yes, your emotions that are unconscious and the ones that you ignore can cause female stress and disease. Again, our health is in direct proportion to our neurological fitness. Stuck emotions and thinking negative thoughts on a regular basis can dis-empower the nervous system and make your organs and hormones unhealthy.

AFFIRMATIONS AND AFFORMATIONS® FOR WOMEN'S WELLNESS

I am very thankful to Dr. Sid Williams, Carolyn Myss, Sondra Ray, Mark Victor Hansen and Dr. Wayne Dyer for helping me understand and live the science of mind/body medicine. As a young Chiropractor who was on her own healing path, their wisdom and guidance has helped me heal my body and my life.

When it comes to the science and truthful power of the use of positive thoughts to correct illness, Louise Hay's books, *You Can Heal Your Life*, 1999, and *Heal Your Body A–Z: The Mental Causes for Physical Illness and the Way to Overcome Them*, 1998 (both Hay House: Carlsbad, CA), have influenced me the most.

Affirmations are high-quality, positive thoughts that we choose to think or say to produce specific desired results. The unconscious mind often interferes with a woman's attempt to use affirmations if she doesn't feel safe, deserving and worthy of receiving her results. Our results are usually in direct proportion to our belief systems. If a woman does not believe she is worthy of, safe to, or deserving of producing whatever she is affirming she will not achieve a high level of success of healing her body or her life with the use of affirmations.

Afformations® a new word not yet in dictionaries are high-quality empowering, positive **questions** that we choose to ask ourselves to produce a specific desired result (created by Noah St. John in his The Great Little book of Afformations® and you can find more information at www.NoahStJohn.com). The latest research states that the brain will always move quickly toward answering questions. Women need to become conscious of how many negative statements, beliefs and disempowering questions they allow themselves to think and feel. Once a woman becomes conscious of her thoughts, she can choose to relax and choose positive Affirmations followed by empowering questions (Afformations®).

In my experience as a doctor, I have found that most people need to convince themselves that it is safe to create bliss and joy both consciously and unconsciously. When one uses affirmations the fearful subconscious tries to block the positive from becoming a reality. Using empowering Afformations® is a wonderful way of helping people relax and feel safe when they are working on their affirmations. Affirmations is a familiar technique and Afformations® is new.

When working with empowering questions, it's important to not answer the question.

Remember to breathe and to stay open to the universe and the parts of your brain that will attract to you the results you are seeking. My advice is to continue doing your affirmations and to add empowering questions if you seek emotional fitness.

The information in the following list of Female Problems and the Affirmations for helping heal these problems were inspired by Louise Hay. The brilliant essence of her work, combined with my own healing and my 32 years as an intuitive Chiropractor, have influenced me to modify her words to fit the needs of my female patients. I am grateful to Louise Hay for leading the pathway of positive affirmations for diseases, and want to honor her for creating this accurate approach to women's wellness that is explained in the following pages.

The following is a list of female problems with positive Affirmations (healing statements) followed by Afformations® (empowering questions) that increase holistic feminine fitness.

Problem

The lumbar spine, (lower back vertebrae) is out of place and interfering with nerves that control the health in a woman's body. Many women hold fear, anger and resentment of abuse in the lower spine. Others feel a lack of support in their lives with or without back pain. For healing affirm:

Affirmations

It is safe for me to release my past and to love myself!

I am sexually innocent, and I am always safe.

I am loved, lovable and full of love.

It is now safe for sexual love and feeling great to be followed by more and more sexual love and bliss!

I am a sexual blessing!

I am now willing for it to be safe to receive support!

Afformations®

Breathe and ask these questions. *(Remember not to answer them.)*

Why am I happily enjoying releasing my past and loving myself?

Why am I sexually innocent?

Why am I always sexually safe?

How am I loved, lovable and full of love?

Why is great divine sexual love always followed by more great divine sexual love?

How am I a sexual blessing?

Why am I safe and receiving divine sexual, loving support?

Why am I happily enjoying receiving support?

Problem

Pain in the lower back. The lower back and the sacral area (tail bone) can be holding on to a time when a woman might have lost her power and is where she might be holding anger. The woman's sacrum holds her uterus in alignment. Anger can twist the pelvis and tip the uterus and cause female distress and disease.

Affirmations

It is now safe to feel powerful and in control! I now take back control of my body and my life.

I am now willing to feel safe and to easily and freely release all that I no longer need. My feminine powers are safe and heal others.

I am worthy and deserving of feeling that I am the power and the authority in my life!

I now easily and effortlessly release the past and deserve to claim my greatness now.

Afformations®

Breathe and ask these questions. (*Remember not to answer them.*)

Why am I happily enjoying feeling safe, powerful and in control?

Why am I enjoying releasing all that I do not need? How am I the power and authority in my life?

Why are my feminine powers now safe?

Why is it easy to release the past and claim my greatness now?

Problem

Malfunction of the pituitary gland. When a woman holds her breath and clenches her jaw she can cause pressure on the bones that hold the pituitary in place. Cranial stress can cause hormonal imbalances.

Affirmations

I am now willing to control my thoughts.

I deserve to have my mind and body in perfect balance.

I can relax and breathe.

I flow with life.

Life now flows easily and peacefully through me.

I am safe now; I am willing to feel safe and healthy now!

Afformations®

Breathe and ask these questions. *(Remember not to answer them.)*

Why am I willing to control my thoughts?

Why am I deserving of balance?

Why am I happily enjoying life to flow easily and peacefully through me?

How am I safe and healthy now?

Why am I happily enjoying the flow of life?

Problem

Painful menstrual cycles. These can be a manifestation of not accepting oneself. When a woman experiences a Chiropractic sacral adjustment she can untip her uterus and release menstrual cramps. Chiropractic can release menstrual cramping most of the time within minutes of an adjustment. To prevent menstrual cramps and to hold Chiropractic adjustments, women must release their negative thoughts and emotions that could be keeping their sacrums out of place.

Affirmations

It is now safe to accept my full power as a woman.

I am now safe to accept all my female functions as normal, natural and beautiful.

It is now safe to love and approve of my sexuality.

I easily and effortlessly forgive myself and my past.

I am now a safe and healed sexual being!

Afformations®

Breathe and ask these questions. *(Remember not to answer them.)*

Why is it now safe to accept my full power as a woman?

Why am I now safe and beautiful?

Why am I enjoying loving and approving of my beautiful sexuality?

How am I a successfully healed sexual being?

Problem

Menopausal discomfort. This can be caused by not feeling good enough, a constant fear of aging and/or a long life of self-rejection. As with all symptoms, we must explore the chemical, emotional and physical components.

Affirmations

I am a sexually honorable great woman!

It is now safe to create balance and peace in all the cycles of my life.

I am now willing to feel good enough as a woman.

I am worthy of blessing my body with my love.

It is now safe to allow others to live their own lessons.

I am deserving of joy.

It is now safe to receive an abundance of sexual blessings.

Afformations®

Breathe and ask these questions. *(Remember not to answer them.)*

Why am I happily enjoying feeling that I am a great woman?

Why am I creating balance, health and peace in all the cycles of my life?

Why am I worthy of my own loving blessings?

Why am I enjoying sexually loving and approving of myself?

Why is it safe to allow others to live their own lessons?

Why am I deserving of sexual joy?

How am I receiving an abundance of sexual blessings?

Problem

Cysts and pain in the ovaries. Ovaries express a woman's creative balance and problems can arise from a lack of honoring the creative spirit. Many women are too busy taking care of everyone else's needs and claim they have no time to nurture their own creative spirit.

Affirmations

It is now safe to honor and balance my creative flow!

I deserve to acknowledge and honor my creative spirit.

I now have enough time to nurture my creative spirit.

I am now willing for it to feel safe to be creative.

Afformations®

Breathe and ask these questions. *(Remember not to answer them.)*

Why am I happily enjoying honoring my creative flow?

Why am I acknowledging my creative spirit?

How am I enjoying enough time to nurture my creative spirit?

Why is it safe to be creative?

Why am I enjoying honoring my creative spirit?

Problem

Malfunctioning of the uterus. The uterus is known as the home of creativity. Pain and disease can come from thoughts and feelings of not belonging in the body. Holding on to a past sexual shame can also cause problems in this area.

Affirmations

I am now willing, and it is safe, to feel at home in my body.

I love and approve of my body and honor its creative flow.

I am a sexual blessing and I am deserving of sexual, loving support.

It is now safe to be open and receptive to loving support!

Afformations®

Breathe and ask these questions. *(Remember not to answer them.)*

Why am I happily enjoying feeling at home in my body?

Why am I loving and approving of my body and honoring its creative flow?

How am I a happy and healed divine sexual blessing?

Why am I deserving of loving support?

Why am I happily enjoying being open and receptive to sexual, loving support?

Problem

Fibroid tumors and cysts. These represent an old pattern and an emotional pain one has not let go of. Many women are often bonded and addicted to the pain of their past experiences. Even though an experience was negative and painful, many women refuse to let go of their past and never look for the reasons why they attracted the pattern. Affirmations to release the patterns that created the problem can help.

Affirmations

I now feel safe to release patterns that created and attracted this experience to me!

I am now willing and deserving to receive only good in my life.

The movies in my mind are beautiful because I choose to safely create them that way.

I love and approve of my sexuality.

Afformations®

Breathe and ask these questions. (*Remember not to answer them.*)

How am I easily forgiving and releasing the patterns that created and attracted this experience to me?

Why am I only creating positive movies in my mind?

Why am I happily enjoying loving and approving of my sexuality?

Why am I enjoying creating positive movies in my mind?

Problem

Pinched nerves in the neck. This area of the body can shut down when we are worrying and trying to control life. The emotional center in the neck shuts down when we are not able to feel or to express our feelings. Many women who suffered physical or emotional oral abuse can be suffering from pinched nerves in their necks. Many women who were told to "shut up" as they grew up might be holding pressure here. Because the neck holds all the nerves for the rest of the body, it is very important to do these affirmations. When we release worry and the need to control life, we relax the neck and balance the nervous system and hormones.

Affirmations

I am now able to express my feelings safely and easily.

It is now safe to express myself.

I safely surrender my will to universal will (to a higher source).

Afformations®

Breathe and ask these questions. *(Remember not to answer them.)*

Why am I happily enjoying expressing my feelings safely and easily?

Why is it safe to express my truth?

How am I happily enjoying surrendering my will to a higher source?

Louise Hay, author of *Heal Your Body,* Hay House: Santa Monica, CA, 1988, has helped me to heal myself and thousands of my patients!
   She states:

   All female problems are a result of self-rejection, rejecting femininity, and rejections of the feminine principle.

   She guides women to rejoice in their femininity. Her work has helped me to understand the emotional reasons for diseases and I recommend this book to all patients.

GENERAL WELLNESS FOR FEMALES

Affirmations

It is now safe to feel deserving and worthy of rejoicing in my female body.

I'm now willing for it to be safe to love my female body.

It is now safe to be a woman and to love my body!

Afformations®

Breathe and ask these questions. *(Remember not to answer them.)*

Why am I rejoicing in my femininity?

Why am I happily enjoying being a great woman?

How do I happily love my female body?

Why am I happily loving being female?

Why is it now safe to enjoy loving being female?

Women's wellness is made up of the joys and pains of their past, their thoughts and emotions in the present and what they believe their future will bring.

I have been a Chiropractor and a holistic healer for over thirty years, and I find Louise Hay's principles to be very accurate for most of my patients. Most of her affirmations end with the thought or prayer that one must love and approve of oneself. It has made me realize how important it is to love oneself and one's body. I highly respect her work and often fine tune her writing to fit my individual patients. It bears repeating: one must feel safe to use affirmations, and feel deserving and worthy of receiving whatever it is one is affirming.

The documentary "The Secret" states that the Universe's Law of Attraction works on our feelings as well as our thoughts.

As a successful Chiropractor who has helped thousands of women, I can truly say that only those who attempt a holistic approach to their health accomplish true healing.

Chiropractic adjustments are holistic and they release chemical, emotional and physical stress. If women want to be totally healthy they must support the Chiropractic adjustment by clearing their emotional reasons for their pain. Some women use Chiropractors as Nature's Midol or Tylenol, and only seek care when they have symptoms. Like the unsuccessful symptomatic medical approach, one will not have long lasting health if one only sees the Chiropractor when they are in pain. If women want to truly heal, they must seek Chiropractors who are experienced in prevention and wellness/greatness care. Women must clear their emotional reasons for their pain if they're going to stop their symptoms from recurring. Holistic feminine fitness happens when women choose Chiropractic preventive wellness visits.

We all have the ability to choose peace. The more a woman chooses peace, the easier her path will be to happier hormones and female greatness!

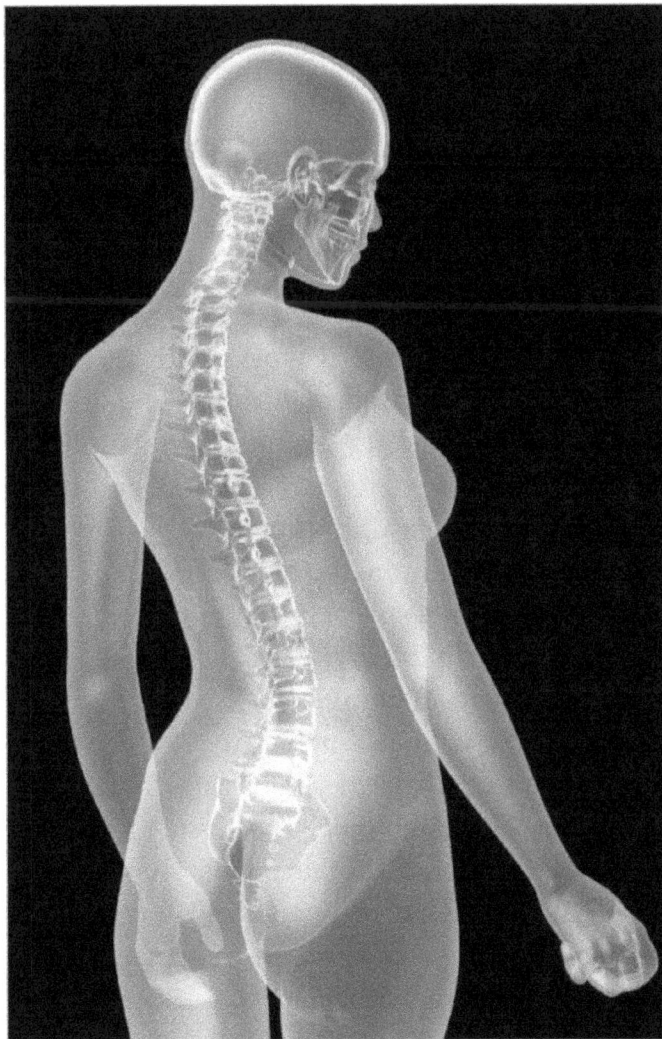

STEP 4

Balance Your Pelvis and Untip Your Uterus

Many women are told that their problems are caused by a tipped uterus, but are never told why it's tipped or how to untip it. They lie on a table, legs in stirrups, and many times are examined and diagnosed from one narrow angle and one viewpoint. This perspective commonly reveals a tipped uterus. Women are given medicine to alleviate their symptoms but are rarely given anything to fix the true cause of their problem. When the drugs no longer hide or help their symptoms, many women are told they need to have their organs removed.

Chiropractic helps the uterus because it works with the neurological (electrical) part of the body that controls its functions. Chiropractic adjustments can physically balance the pelvic bones that are holding the uterus in its improper position. When the uterus is balanced, it is happy, free of nerve pressure and functions well. The balancing of the pelvis and uterus with a Chiropractic adjustment helps many women eliminate their toxic drug intake and often prevents surgery!

I know this might be too simple for you to believe so please look this up in an anatomy book or just look at the picture of the woman's pelvis at the end of this chapter. The sacral uterine ligaments hold the uterus in its place. These ligaments go from the sacrum (tail bone) to the uterus. If the pelvis is twisted, the uterus will also be twisted. If you are having menstrual cramps and the cause is a tipped uterus, simple and safe Chiropractic pelvic adjustments can correct the misalignment of your pelvis and balance your tipped uterus. I have had my

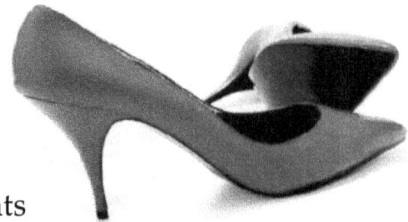

menstrual cramps relieved by Chiropractic adjustments, and have helped thousands of women to experience the joy of a balanced pelvis and a happy uterus.

Wearing high heels, crossing one's legs, standing or sitting on one leg or hip, driving twisted, traumatic births, sexual abuse, congenital malformations, and falls are some of the reasons that can cause the pelvic bones to get twisted and out of balance. Also unsymmetrical sports, exercises, occupational posture and habits can tip the sacrum (pelvic bone) out of balance and cause the uterus to malfunction.

Women need to balance their pelvis and hipbones to experience the bliss of healthy cycles. Wearing high heels can put your uterus in an anterior downward horizontal position. Wearing sensible shoes allows your uterus to stand up straight. High heels can cause your uterus to fight the natural pull of gravity and cause it to cramp when it wants to shed its tissues and bleed.

Do you keep your legs and pelvis twisted in a chair, at the gym, computer, at school, work, or at home? If you are experiencing painful cycles, make some changes and choose to balance your pelvis. Cut down on wearing high heels and give your innate intelligence that runs your uterus the chance to function more efficiently.

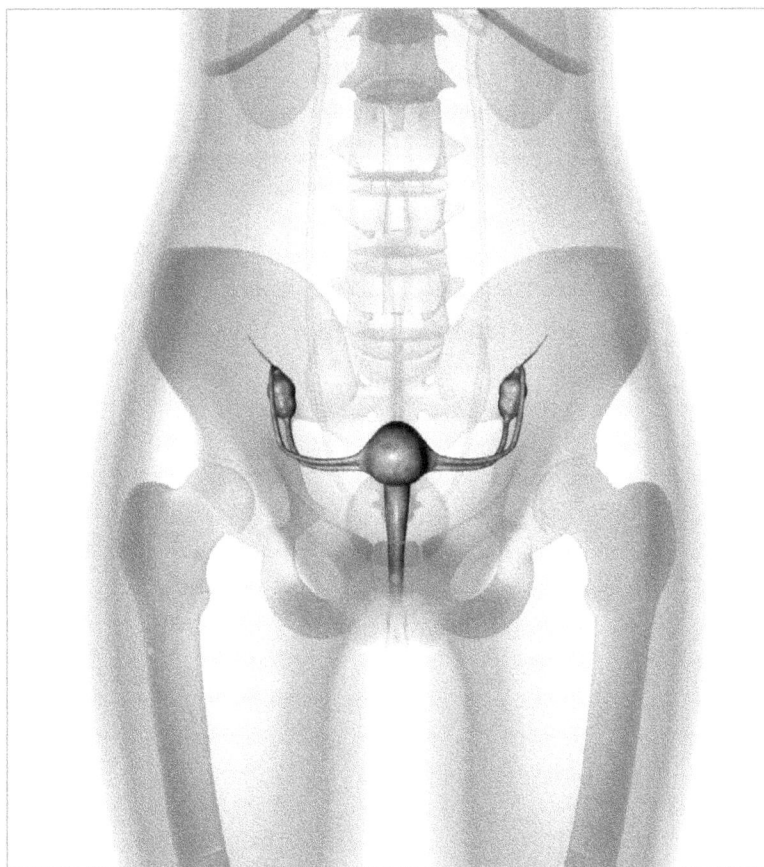

If your car's chassis was out of alignment the tires would continue to wear out. Would you keep buying new tires on your car, or would you be concerned about its alignment and investigate the true reason for your tires having problems? Your hips are the tires of your car (body) and they need to be balanced, healthy and strong to hold your uterus in place. Gentle Chiropractic adjustments balance the hip sockets and pelvic bones so that the uterus can be balanced and healthy. Besides having Chiropractic adjustments, women also need to assume postures that strengthen the pelvis, and limit the time they wear high heels. Some women wear sandals that have a "negative heel" effect that can tip their pelvis and uterus into a backward position. A forward or backward tipped uterus can cause menstrual cramping and other female problems.

Creating balance in the pelvis can help to relieve menstrual cramps, and it can also assist infertile women to become pregnant. During pregnancy, Chiropractic adjustments can help alleviate sinus pressure, headaches, nausea, pain, swelling and numbness. Many women choose Chiropractic during pregnancy and while breast feeding because it can produce results without any harmful drugs. Balancing the pelvis and uterus can also promote easier and safer deliveries. Again, balance is the key to a woman's pelvis and life, and will always produce a healthy effect on the functioning of the uterus. At any age, and all day long, women should keep their bones in healthy positions and not just during a Yoga or a Tai Chi class.

Is looking great and sexy in high heels worth all the side effects of the drugs you might be taking to counteract your unhealthy symptoms or worth the possibility of surgical removal of your female organs?

Please ladies, do not dress your little girls in high heels! It is very important to be balanced especially when growing. Little girls who wear high heels are tipping their pelvis in an unhealthy direction and tipping their uteruses at a very young age.

STEP 5

Practice Spinal Hygiene
All Day Long

You can't brush your spine so keep it in line!

In the previous chapters, I have discussed the fundamental relationships that exist between the nervous system and your health. A fully functioning nervous system is of utmost importance in achieving optimum health. The nervous system controls all cellular activities, including all bodily functions. Your spinal column protects this great system from harm. If you want to be a healthy, successful female, spinal hygiene must become a daily habit.

Spinal hygiene is the daily practice of healing postures that allows your nervous system to stay healthy and fit. Take out that mental dental floss again. Stay open to change and new ways of healing yourself. Poor posture impedes the messages flowing between the brain and the body.

If you want to be a great and healthy female, become aware of your spinal habits. Most women understand the value of good dental hygiene, but many are not aware that practicing daily spinal hygiene is vital for a healthy life. Ignoring spinal hygiene is as damaging to the nervous system as forgetting about dental hygiene and letting your teeth decay. Obviously you cannot use a toothbrush on your spine.

By becoming aware of poor posture habits and correcting them, you can dramatically improve your level of neurological fitness. Practicing daily spinal hygiene will keep the spinal column aligned so the flow of information between your nervous system and the rest of your body remains open and unobstructed.

If people practiced spinal hygiene and visited their Chiropractor more often, they would be less dependent on prescription drugs and many surgical procedures would be unnecessary. Visits to a Chiropractor and daily spinal hygiene keep you neurologically fit in much the same way daily dental hygiene and regular visits to your dentist help you maintain healthy teeth.

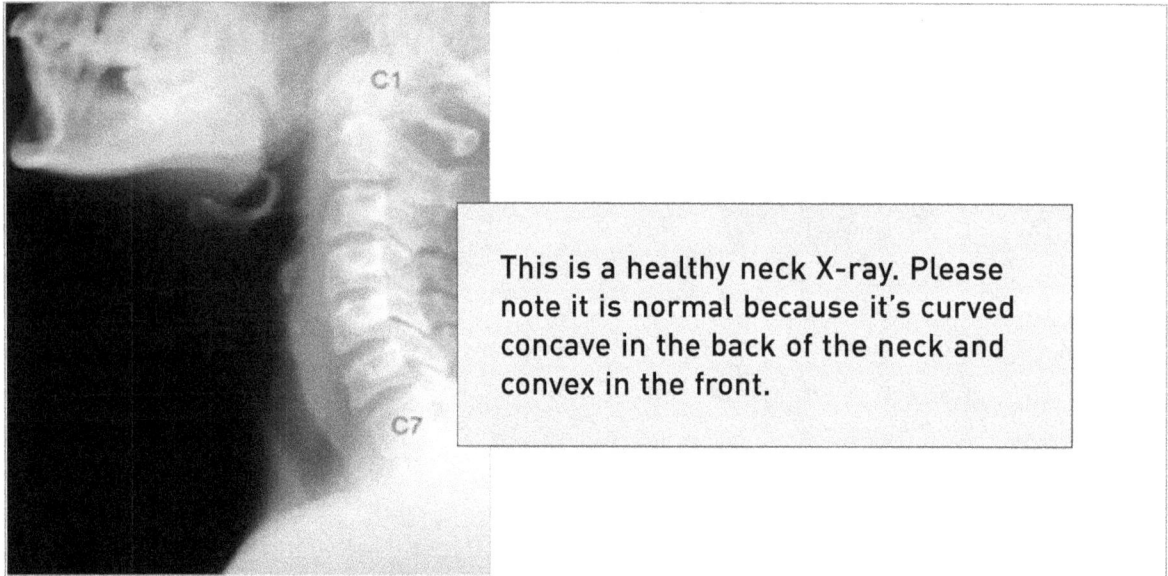

This is a healthy neck X-ray. Please note it is normal because it's curved concave in the back of the neck and convex in the front.

Using the Computer

Where is your computer monitor located? If the position of your monitor requires you to look down or to the side, then change it. Place books or a block of wood under the screen to raise it. You'll be more creative, and your brain function, productivity, and memory will improve. Also, remember to breathe while working at the computer. Holding your breath and/or clenching your jaw when you are concentrating on a task can inhibit the flow of oxygen to your brain and your body.

If you are working on a laptop, sit up straight, raise the screen to eye level and buy a wireless keyboard. If you don't use a wireless keyboard, and you raise your computer up, you will be holding your shoulders too high which can pinch the nerves in your shoulders, elbows, and carpal tunnel bones. Keep your eyes focused on the center of the monitor

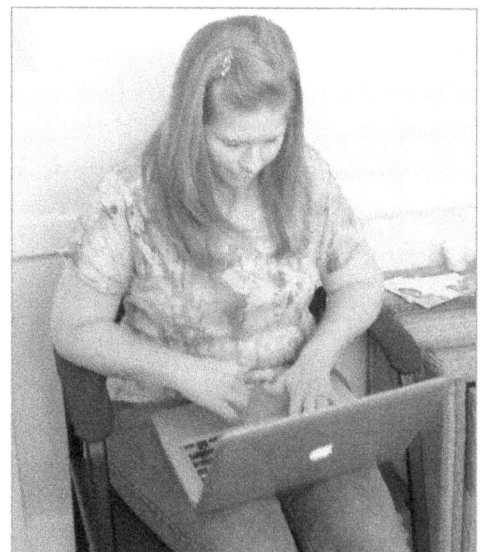

Unhealthy laptop posture

rather than the bottom. You can accomplish this by simply scrolling the page up often. To determine the correct height of your computer monitor, bring your shoulders back and line your ears up in the same plane. Keep your chin up and away from your throat. Ask someone to check your height at the computer after you have chosen a healthy posture. While using your computer, check your breathing pattern often and relax while squeezing your shoulders back. Make sure that both feet are planted evenly on the floor and you are sitting evenly on both buttocks. Improve your spinal posture and you will increase your female greatness!

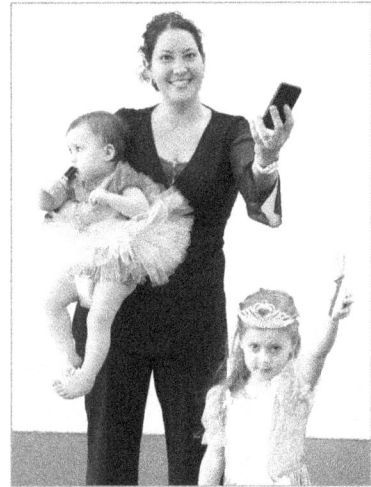

Looking Up is Healthy!

Reading

This is one of the most difficult postures to correct. If you hold the book on your lap and look down for extended periods of time you stress your nervous system. Use several pillows under your elbows to keep the book up to eye level while sitting on a couch or chair. If you are seated at a desk, bookstands can hold the book up. Chair desks keep the book up at eye level; they are expensive. An alternate solution is to use a music stand, to hold the book in an upright position.

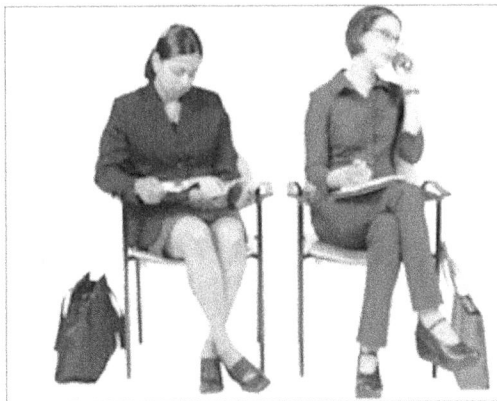

Set a timer and take short breaks every fifteen minutes or so. Taking short breaks can undo the damage that might be caused by the downward position of head and chin when you are reading when seated. An excellent Spinal Hygiene practice would be to get up often and lean against an open door frame. Stand up straight and pull your shoulders backward and do the backstroke. Lean your head and spine against the doorframe to support your head and body. Begin with the backwards breaststroke (arms moving back together) followed by the backstroke (alternating arms). This will alleviate stress caused by holding your head down while reading or studying. Remember to look up and breathe through these exercises in the doorway. Of course, using these swimming strokes in a pool is even more beneficial.

Reclining while reading in bed using two or three pillows to prop up your head causes the chin to rest down on the throat and chest and puts stress on the neck. The neck bones need to be concave at the back and the chin needs to be in a neutral position if you want to be healthy. If you must read in bed, take a small towel and roll it up to the size of the nape of your neck. Place the roll under your neck so the neck is arched and your chin is facing up rather than down. Hold the book up to eye level with one hand and alternate hands as they tire. The neck is the most important part of the spine because all nerves must pass through it to communicate with the rest of the body. If you find yourself looking down a lot, keep these tips in mind and remember to take frequent breaks.

Texting and Video Games

A major problem in our society right now that is harming the health of women and children is the unhealthy posture of texting and game playing! Most hold their heads downwards while their shoulders are hunched forward, which puts an enormous pressure on the brain stem and spinal nerves. The one sided texting posture when one is using only one hand keeps the head tipped down on one side and is the most harmful to the nervous system. Raise the cell phone up to eye level and pull your shoulders back to prevent pinching the nerves in your neck. At first, texting with your head in a neutral position and holding the phone up to eye level will be difficult and feel awkward but it's good for your health. Maintaining good spinal hygiene will boost your female health and success. Young children spending a lot of time with video games usually have their heads downwards and are creating pressure on their brain stems.

Talking on the Phone

Another posture that may be affecting your energy is the position of your head when using the phone. If you want to create more energy, hormonal balance, a healthier memory, and holistic neurological fitness, refrain from keeping your head and neck in a twisted position when talking on the phone. Alternate your listening ear and try keeping your head in a neutral position. This will help to balance your brainstem. Using a headset can keep your neck and cranium balanced and in proper position. A Blue Tooth also helps, but many people tip their skull to the side of the Blue Tooth because of the weight on that side.

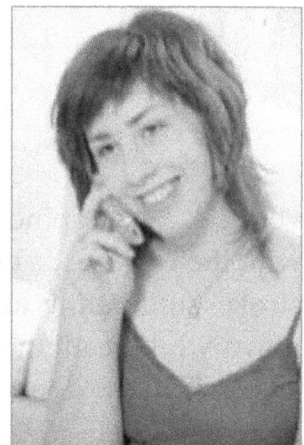

Breathe when it is your time to listen. Breathing will help you relax. When you receive negative information you most likely clench your jaw, and your head might be twisted which causes pressure on your nerves. Remind yourself to breathe, to unclench your jaw, to tip your chin up, and to squeeze your shoulders back when hearing upsetting news. By remembering these tips, you will be practicing spinal hygiene.

Writing

We use our dominant eye and ear when we are writing, cutting, using the phone or cleaning. This causes the head to tilt to one side. If you must write for an extended period of time, take some breaks and stretch your neck and head to the opposite side. Try to write with your head tilted the opposite way. It might feel strange at first, but it's better for spinal hygiene. Writing is a great activity to realize how one-sided you've become. Stretch your neck in both directions to enjoy more energy.

Driving

Many of us drive in a "turtle position." We sink our necks and heads into our "shells" and raise our shoulders up too high. Squeeze your shoulders backward, drop and relax them, and place your hands in the middle or at the bottom of the wheel whenever possible. Breathe, keep your shoulders dropped, raise your chin, unclench your jaw and try to relax when you are driving. Be especially conscious of this in traffic. Your left buttock muscle, hip, knee, and foot should mirror the right leg. By doing this you will be sitting balanced, thus preventing spinal and pelvic problems, and uneven pressure on your joints.

Remember, you can't brush your spine . . . so keep it in line!

Exercising

Many sports require asymmetrical postures. Participating in these sports causes a twisting of the spine in one direction which causes an imbalance in the spinal column. After tennis, golf, or bowling, or any one-sided sport, it's a good idea to stretch and twist in the opposite direction in order to bring your spine back into balance. When exercising at the gym remember to keep your head up. Many people pull their chins down when lifting weights or doing sit-ups which causes harm to the nervous system. People who exercise often may look physically fit, but not be healthy on the inside. Over the past 32 years I have x-rayed many body builders. Many of their x-rays reveal that they have much older internal bodies than their outward physical appearance. These body builders may actually be increasing their internal weakness by lifting weights without assuming the proper posture.

When lifting weights, it's important that your neck is positioned correctly or you could suffer injuries, which might cause internal aging. Do you want to look just physically great or do you want to be totally fit?

Make spinal hygiene a habit by assuming proper posture whenever you are exercising. This is very important, especially if you are lifting weights. Keep your chin up, which means you should not be reading while using the treadmill, stair stepper, elliptical or stationary bike unless you can support the book at eye level at the same time.

Sit-ups is another exercise that can destroy the natural curve of the neck. Keep your neck arched and support it with a towel (or your hands) when performing abdominal exercises. Remember that total fitness is more than just having "washboard abs" (abdominals). Total fitness is health on all levels. If you are not using the proper posture(s), you can interfere with the nerves to organs; affect your attitude, your memory, your energy and your cycles.

Now that you've become familiar with the Spinal Posture Secrets that promote neurological fitness, look at the chart in the previous chapter. You will see why your posture is so important. Your body's functions depend on the nervous system. The spine, pelvis, and cranium are bones that protect the nerves and hold them in place. The cervical curve (neck area) is concave in the back. So now you can see why it is important to monitor your posture and practice daily spinal hygiene.

Your body is a miracle. Millions of functions are happening inside of you without you even thinking about them. The nervous system is extremely sensitive to physical stress. You need to reduce this stress so you can be healthy, fully-functioning and living at your highest potential.

Chiropractic, like dentistry, is a team effort and needs daily spinal hygiene to have great results.

Reduce Toxic Thoughts and Foods That Can Cause Hormonal Imbalances

Are you hormonal or just toxic?

You are what you eat! Many women experience the effects of stomach stress, liver toxicity, and neurological dysfunction, and have been trained to blame their monthly "cyclic" symptoms on their hormones, genetics, or just their sexuality!

As a Chiropractor who has helped thousands of women during their premenstrual, menstrual, postmenstrual, prenatal, postnatal, breast feeding, premenopausal, menopausal and postmenopausal cycles, I have found that when you limit your junk food, and take great care of your spine and nervous system, your hormonal cycles and the rest of your body will be healthier and happier.

I have personally experienced cyclic female stress whenever I was overeating and binging on junk food. When my diet was healthy and I was diligent with my spinal hygiene, I did not suffer hormonal stress.

When you eat too many toxic foods your Innate Intelligence becomes chemically toxic, slows down and the doctor inside of you goes to sleep. When the nervous system doesn't get its proper nutrients and the digestive system doesn't function at its optimum, your hormones can, and will, swing out of balance.

Many women suffer from low blood sugar just before their menstrual periods or when they are ovulating. Women who "pig out" and binge on sugar suffer from extreme low blood sugar at the time their hormones are fluctuating. This is one of the reasons premenstrual syndrome (PMS) causes women to be sad, angry or depressed. To raise their blood sugar levels and to help themselves feel better women crave and overeat candy. Many patients I have helped with this have had to be very careful with their diets during the whole month to prevent low blood sugar dips during their cycles.

Besides causing emotional stress, this drop in blood sugar causes headaches, migraines, and sometimes dizziness. Eating protein snacks and eating small meals six times a day can usually balance blood sugar and prevent mood swings.

Balancing blood sugar levels can also help alleviate morning sickness. Nausea can also be caused when cranial bones and the upper neck area are out of place. I have seen thousands of women get rid of their morning sickness with Chiropractic adjustments and by balancing their blood sugar.

Balancing blood sugar levels can also reduce menopausal symptoms. Hot flashes, depression, anxiety, swelling, and brain fog, are an indication that a woman is chemically out of balance. Another thing a woman can do to alleviate hot flashes is to reduce the amount of caffeine, alcohol, preservatives and/or dyes in her diet. A major culprit that sabotages female health is the willingness to believe in, and follow, fad diets. This often leads to toxicity, and makes women neurologically impaired and hormonally sick. We are greatly influenced by mass media and follow nutrition fads that are not always in our best interest. The biggest example is the promotion of the deadly no-fat or low-fat diet. The misperception is that eating fat can make you fat or cause you to have a stroke or heart attack. So like sheep many women follow the masses and choose no-fat or low-fat foods. The United States leads the world in obesity, and has one of the highest rates of heart attacks and strokes while remaining on this ridiculous diet.

We were told not to eat eggs, and definitely not to eat the yellow of the egg because of its fat content. Research has proven that the organic egg is one of the most nutritious foods we can eat, but only if we eat the whole egg. Eating only egg whites does not prevent obesity nor heart disease. The newest research about the egg is that it raises the good cholesterol, totally opposite to what we have been taught. The whole organic egg has the perfect balance of the omega oils we expect to get from fish oil pills.

Because we are afraid to eat fat, we are left with stiff joints, slower working brains, hormonal imbalances, and nervous systems that are starving. **The nervous system needs fat to survive.**

We have starved the very system that controls our health and our hormones. When I was growing up, people took the skins off fish to prevent heart disease; now everyone pops fish oil pills to heal themselves from this horrendous nutritional mistake.

We were told for years not to eat nuts because of their fat content, and now we are told they reduce cholesterol and heart disease. We were told not to eat butter but to eat "plastic" margarine because of the fat in butter. Now we know butter is better. They are now producing butter pills to increase the health of the circulatory system.

We were told to use sun block or not to go in the sun. Now we are told that we are vitamin D deficient, and sun block stops the healthy sunrays that create magical vitamin D. Vitamin D helps our bones and immune systems. The pharmaceutical companies are getting rich on producing vitamin D pills. The sad fact is that the yellow of the egg has the magical ability to take the sun's rays and convert them into vitamin D. If you don't have enough cholesterol in your system you cannot make vitamin D from the sun.

To further confuse you, the French are some of the thinnest people in the world and they eat lots of cream, sugar, butter and white flour. They enjoy and chew their food without guilt, and they are thinner and healthier than we are.

We take better care of our cars then we do our bodies! Cars get aligned in their first year of life. We drive an extra mile to get better gas. We know that our cars' alignment and what we feed them is directly proportional to how well they will function. The same holds true for our bodies. We are what we eat, and our health is directly proportional to the nourishment we choose. The alignment of our spines and the health of our nervous systems determine how well we digest our food.

Chemistry matters if you want to go from wellness to greatness. Keep healthy fats and oils in your diet if you want to enjoy a healthy brain, balanced hormones and a highly functioning nervous system. It's always better to eat the food that has what you need in it, than to take a pill that claims to have the same properties. Your body assimilates the food better than the pill. Our bodies sometimes cannot even digest the coatings on the pills that we pop, and the coatings can be toxic to our systems. We are spending millions of dollars on medicine and vitamins yet our health has not improved.

Vitamins should be from actual food sources and not be synthetic. The cheaper brands found in wholesale stores, drug stores, and supermarkets have more poisons in them then those sold in health food stores. Read the labels on your vitamins, and if there are words that you don't recognize, don't buy the vitamins. Spend a little more money on healthy foods and vitamins, and you'll get less additives, preservatives, pesticides and poisons. Less toxicity creates healthier female cycles.

Eat small meals regularly and drink plenty of water. Your brain needs glucose and hydration to function. Living in a dehydrated state or with high or low blood sugar levels can cause "brain fog" and memory loss. If you want to be a great and healthy woman you must balance your chemistry. Do not skip meals, and remember to drink plenty of water.

To ensure good female health, aim at drinking half your body weight in ounces of water a day. There are many opinions on this matter. The important thing to remember is that if you want to boost your memory, and enjoy good health, stay hydrated. Many women are suffering because they're living on coffee and not drinking enough water. Rule of thumb: for every cup of coffee you need to add an additional three cups of water to break even and keep your kidneys happy. Another fad to watch out for is the so-called need for alkaline water. Research has been showing that cancer thrives in an acid environment. Ladies, please test your pH before you decide that you need to be more alkaline. We need to be balanced to be healthy and in ten years from now they might be telling us the opposite information. Many women are too alkaline to begin with and could have stomach problems if they become more alkaline. Again, think balance and be leery of fads.

Slight dehydration can cause your lower back muscles to be toxic and tight. This can pinch nerves and cause back pain, hip pain, knee pain and lower limbs to be painful or numb.

Ironically, dehydration can contribute to high blood pressure. Many women taking high blood pressure pills that contain a diuretic may be creating a slight state of dehydration and the constant need for high blood pressure pills. Check with your medical doctor to find out the true reason for your high blood pressure. Is it due to a malfunctioning of your cardiovascular system, your urinary system, or your nervous system?

Drinking diet sodas to hydrate is not a good idea because the chemicals in them retard the brain. Statistics have shown that the artificial sweetener, aspartame, found in diet sodas has caused people to stay fat, and has increased auto immune diseases. Aspartame has increased the incidences of convulsions and seizures, multiple sclerosis (MS) and lupus. Diet sodas can keep belly fat levels high and are very addictive. If you have to have a soda once in a while, choose the real old-fashioned sugar kind. Read all food labels. "No sugar added," or "light" could mean the food was sweetened with toxic chemicals. Stevia and agave are healthy choices for sweeteners.

So are you hormonal or just toxic?

The latest research states that raw organic fruits and vegetables contain all the natural antioxidants and anti-inflammatory ingredients we need to prevent heart disease, diabetes and cancer. We need 9 to 12 portions of raw, organic fruits and vegetables a day to stay healthy and to prevent memory loss. If you cannot eat this much, find healthy fruit and vegetable capsules, juices and powders in the health food store, but remember the real food is always the better choice.

You cannot be neurologically fit nor have happy, healthy hormones, if you do not feed yourself properly. Think of yourself as an expensive car that needs great gasoline to function at a high level. Reduce the amount of junk food, increase the intake of nutritious food, and you will keep your brain and hormones balanced, happy, smart and healthy.

Information on soybeans, caffeine and eggs are constantly changing. Previous information told us that soy could help to prevent cancer and now we read that can cause breast cancer. What are we to believe? Do we eat eggs or not? Are dark chocolate and wine really good for everyone? Nutritional experts change their minds daily; something that you read today can be false tomorrow.

Many women experience hot flashes after drinking wine and eating chocolate. I have taken care of hundreds of women who confessed to me that their pre-menstrual blues and headaches and premenopausal and menopausal hot flashes disappeared when their diets were healthy and balanced. These same women also realized that binging on wine, sugar, meat, coffee, pizza and packaged or frozen foods brought back their uncomfortable symptoms.

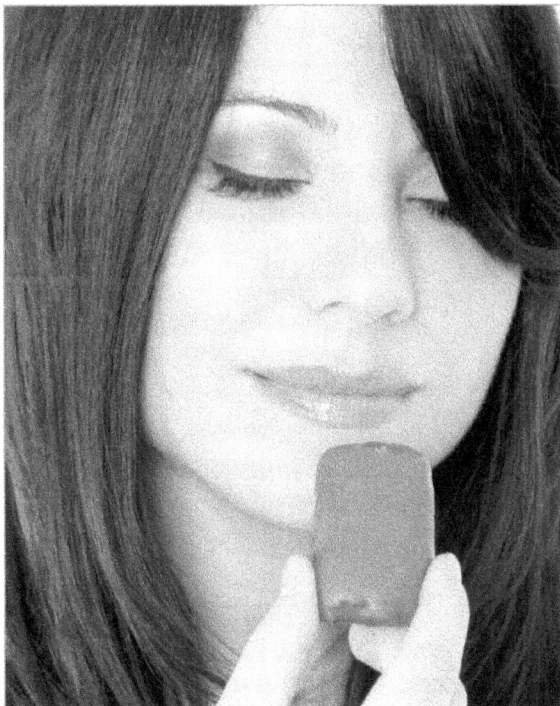

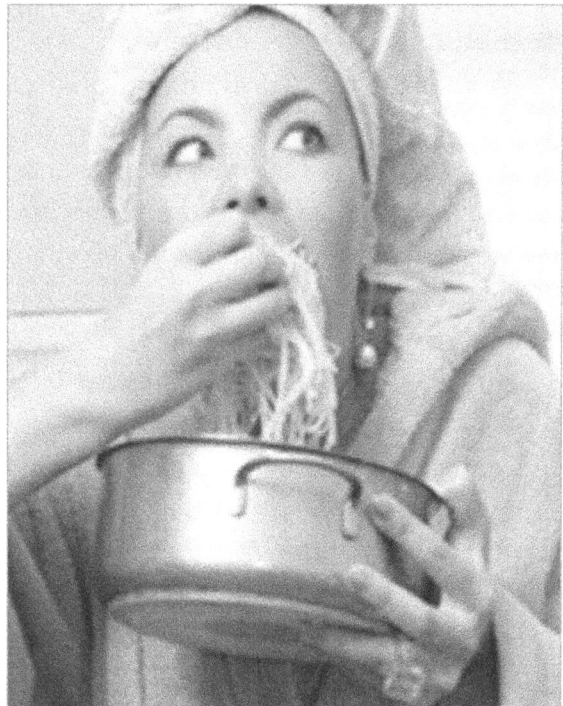

Which woman represents how you feel when you are eating? Are you rushing or feeling guilty? Are you taking the time to chew your food? Are you allowing your mealtime to be a pleasurable peaceful experience?

Are you enjoying your food, or are you in a state of worry, anger or guilt when eating? (The French take the time to enjoy their food.)

Choosing peace, balance and happiness are emotional keys to a healthy digestive system and a healthy female life. It's not always what you eat, but how your digestive system processes the food. How you are digesting life can be directly related to how you digest your food. **If you are having problems digesting your food, your stomach and liver can become toxic, and you might not have any symptoms other than unhappy unbalanced hormones.**

Eat as many organic foods as you can afford. Buy meat, chicken, milk products and eggs that are free of hormones and antibiotics. Reduce the amount of processed foods, and increase the amount of raw organic fresh fruits and vegetables. Increase the amount of good oils and fats from healthy fish, nuts and vegetables. Reduce the amount of farmed fish that have been fed toxic dyes to enhance color.

So, are you hormonal or toxic? I have seen hundreds of women banish their menstrual cramps and hot flashes with Chiropractic care and by reducing their intake of pizza, alcohol, sugar and caffeine. I have also seen hundreds of women prevent their female discomfort with Chiropractic care alone without changing their diets and can eat whatever they want. The differences in these two groups of women are usually their attitudes and the amount of toxic thoughts and feelings they hold on to.

Women of the world, try to take extra breaths before you eat; relax and calm down. Release the past, accept the now, and expect great joy before you eat. Take the time to thank the food and bless whatever goes in your mouth. Your thoughts and postures before, during and after eating create your level of nutritional fitness. Having negative thoughts about the food can be worse for you than the actual chemistry of the food.

If you decide to eat it, bless it, chew it and enjoy it!

Nutrition fads change like the wind. Do not be like a little lamb that follows the flock and believes in fad diets. By choosing not to follow the "norm", you will be healthier than those that blindly eliminate foods which are vital to their health. Beware of any diet that is short on healthy oils, fats, proteins and carbohydrates. They are all necessary for women's wellness and holistic fitness.

The so-called preventative diets for heart disease and cancer have failed to reduce these diseases. When they told us not to eat the saturated fat from the coconut they also told us that you could eat 4 to 6 ounces of steak. Now coconut oil is being touted for its healing properties for heart disease. Mass media, drug companies, and the dairy and meat lobbies spend millions of dollars promoting food fallacies.

If you are constipated and your stomach and liver are toxic, there is a good chance that you will have pain and misery during your female cycles. Like your thoughts and your posture, you can control your diet.

If you have hot flashes and know you have a great diet, please visit a (holistic)

Chiropractor. Chiropractic is always holistic but not all Chiropractors practice authentic, principled Chiropractic. If your Chiropractor only wants to see you when you have symptoms or are in pain you might not be in the right office. Remember the symptomatic approach belongs to the medical profession, and real Chiropractic goes beyond symptoms and on to greater levels of vitality, health, and fitness.

Over the past thirty years, I have found that women who have rounded shoulders, and poor posture create pinched nerves in their neck and upper back, and suffer the most hormonal stress. When you sleep try not to tuck your head down over your throat and do not allow your shoulders to fall forward. When you have shoulder and neck pressure, you can have a pinched nerve to the digestive system. Lying on your side at night rolled up in the fetal position can put pressure on the nerves to the stomach and may cause nighttime hot flashes. Another problem that I have found with females that can cause postural stress and result in digestive and hormonal stress is the clutching and hugging of pocket books and purses. Relax your shoulders and hold them backwards while carrying a purse and at night when you are sleeping if you want to increase nutritional fitness and female health.

Chiropractors who are gentle and specific can adjust your nervous system; relieve hot flashes, and all other hormonal problems. Chiropractic helps the female body to live up to its potential. However, it is up to women to change their sleeping habits and to choose healthy postures, thoughts, and diets during the day, so that their Chiropractic adjustments will hold while they are asleep. Our levels of nutritional fitness are directly proportional to our levels of holistic neurological fitness.

The road from Women's Wellness to Greatness is an inside job and a personal choice.

STEP 7

Choose Holistic Feminine Fitness and Enjoy Total Health

I f women want to enjoy holistic feminine fitness, they need to choose natural alternatives. This could mean choosing the opposite of what is popular with their friends and family. It will require courage to be an independent thinker and to choose to act out of the box.

People in the United States spend the most money on healthcare in the world, yet they rank only 37th in worldwide health.

Let's look at the facts:

- They eat the least amount of healthy fats, consume the most processed no or low fat foods, yet are the fattest, and hold the record for the most heart disease.

- They have the most cancer insurance and cancer awareness in the world, yet have the most cancer.

- They give their children no-fat/skim milk to prevent obesity, yet have the fattest kids in the world. The children of the United States are not as smart or healthy as other children who drink whole milk. They are missing the necessary fats that would enable them to function at their highest potential.

- They are the most vaccinated country in the world, yet have the highest rates of Autism, Alzheimer's, cancer and children's (so-called) asthma. They lead the world in the overuse of antibiotics and steroids.

Something is wrong in this country, and I believe it's because the health insurers and the government refuse to look at the whole person. The United States takes care of their population with "crisis insurance."

All of the insurance companies I am contracted with pay me only if someone is in pain. If a person wants to prevent disease or maintain high energy and holistic fitness, it becomes their "out of pocket" expense and not the insurance company's responsibility. People are paying a lot for health insurance in the United States, but they are not receiving wellness care or true healthcare. Holistic feminine fitness needs to be incorporated into the healthcare system so women are no longer powerless. Holistic feminine fitness happens when a woman decides to balance and enjoy her mind, body, and spirit, at home and at work. It happens when she chooses to be healthy in her soul and her spirit! If women do not think and act holistically with their bodies and lives they will end up like their parents who take an average of five medications a day and possibly have had more than three surgeries.

If you do not want to be one of the USA's horrible statistics on health you must make up your own mind and make healthy choices that are not popular and go in the opposite direction of unhealthy fads.

Women must choose a natural approach to life and health if they want holistic fitness, health and greatness. Many women choose nutrition, some choose exercise and others choose mind control to try and reach a healthy state of being. If women want to achieve a high level of greatness, they must make sure that they are healing themselves on *all* levels. If you leave out any parts of holistic fitness, you might be taking a risk with your health.

Chiropractors are doctors who help the female body do what it was created to do. Chiropractors help women heal from within, and enrich the blood and nervous supply to all the female organs and glands. When a woman receives a specific neurological "Chiropractic tune-up," her emotional, chemical, physical, and spiritual being is attended to and she can enjoy a high state of feminine holistic fitness. A Chiropractor is a woman's best friend from the time she is born to the time she dies.

It is still not popular to visit a Chiropractor to increase the neurological supply to the organs, and to remove the real cause of most health problems. Chiropractic and the natural "magic" that women are born with is still a secret in our society, as is spinal hygiene and holistic neurological fitness. "Big Pharma" (unethical pharmaceutical companies), does not want you to know how to heal yourself without drugs or surgery. Their misinformation and the toxic overuse of drugs have made women powerless about their health. They want you to believe that Chiropractic is only good for back pain and, if you believe this old-fashioned, biased opinion of Chiropractic and live in their "symptomatic" world, they will stay rich.

Women have been misguided about healthy fats that are needed to prevent cancer, heart disease, osteoporosis and hormonal balance. Some pills manufactured for osteoporosis can cause the jawbone to de-mineralize. Women are still taking these medications to strengthen their bones, knowing their jawbones are negatively affected. The jaw is very close to the brain! Is Big Pharma trying to dismantle your cranial bones and mess up your brains? Why would you choose to take a pill to prevent osteoporosis in some bones that is known to weaken your jaw? Please read the side effects if you take osteoporosis medication.

Cholesterol-lowering medication and too little natural sunlight can cause vitamin D deficiencies and can impede the metabolizing of calcium. Who benefits if you are not eating healthy fats, staying out of the sun and are deficient in Vitamin D?

Big Pharma is getting richer daily selling women vitamin D pills.

Unfortunately we are living at a time when women are being told that toxic vaccines are safe when they are pregnant and breastfeeding. I believe that we all need to educate ourselves before we choose vaccines. In the past, pregnant and breastfeeding women have been instructed to choose a natural path whenever possible. It is common knowledge that at this precious special time baby and mama's body are one and not separate. Fear tactics are being used by mass media and "Big Pharma" to scare pregnant and breast feeding women into taking vaccines. Since most of my body was paralyzed from an allergic reaction to a vaccine I often get asked which vaccine was the culprit. My answer is that I took the paralyzing one as it does not matter which one; anyone of them can paralyze you. Below is a list of ingredients found in most vaccines.

Gelatin, Formaldehyde, Aluminum, Sorbitol, Sodium Chloride, Egg Protein, Cow Serum, Human Albumin, Phenoxyethanol, Polysorbate 80, Antibiotics, Thimerosal (Mercury), MSG, GMOs, hormones from infected cows, chickens and monkeys, cross-bred bacteria from animals, mosquitoes and diseased humans.

These poisons are very toxic for pregnant women, breastfeeding women or anyone else to receive. Please visit the National Vaccine Information Center and Educate-beforeyouvaccinate.com for more information.

Chiropractic, spinal hygiene and neurological fitness hold the key to natural immunity and authentic female greatness.

When is the best time to receive this kind of women's holistic health care? The very best time is in the womb. Future generations can be healthier if all women are balanced and adjusted by a Chiropractor when they are pregnant. When next? The next best time for women to receive holistic care is when they are first born. Infants can have birth trauma and should be checked by a Chiropractor soon after they are born.

Newborns and children suffer from problems that can be alleviated naturally if their parents take a holistic approach to healthcare. Breast feeding problems, headaches, colic, sleep problems, allergies, headaches, weak immune systems, asthma, autism, ADD and ADHD, learning problems, hyperactivity, and developmental delays all respond quickly to Chiropractic care.

If you were not seen by a Chiropractor when you were in the womb or shortly after birth, relax, you are never too old to receive holistic feminine care. As long as you are breathing and own a pelvis, cranial bones and a spine, you can enjoy neurological tune- ups, like a grand piano!

You were born with a miraculous intelligence that is always regenerating and rejuvenating its cells. Holistic feminine fitness can be achieved when a woman works on healing, strengthening and balancing her mind, body, soul and spirit. Holistic feminine fitness happens when a woman pays attention to her nervous system and reduces stress on all levels. Healing postures, healthy foods and happy thoughts are all part of holistic feminine fitness. You were born for health and to create a joyous life. This vital information must be passed on to other females, and is important for future generations. Choose holistic and know that all parts of you are important to love and to take care of.

STEP 8

Embrace the ChiroChi® Lifestyle All Day Long

Many women are taking Yoga classes and are experiencing its health benefits of spiritual, emotional and physical bliss. Yoga taps into the magic of healing spinal positions, a relaxed mind and the power of one's breath. Some women do Yoga three hours a week, some an hour a day.

Many women are also choosing Tai Chi classes. Like Yoga, Tai Chi works with healing postures, slow movements and the magic of one's breath. Through its circulation of breath and slow flowing dance like movements, women are experiencing healing on spiritual, emotional and physical levels. Tai Chi is becoming very popular and some women take classes three hours a week, some an hour a day.

CHIROCHI®

ChiroChi® is similar to Yoga and Tai Chi because it also concentrates on the healing of the mind, body and spirit using spinal healing postures, conscious, connected circular breathing and emotional/spiritual fitness. ChiroChi is the conscious choice to be a Tai Chi/Yoga Master all day long and not just at a class or when watching a video.

I am known as a "ChiroSpirit." I teach the true principles of Chiropractic! ChiroChi is the spirit of Chiropractic and is found on every page of this book. The first three letters of Chiropractic are Chi! Chi (Qi) means vital force, energy and life force in the far and Middle East. ChiroChi is the conscious practice of choosing healing spinal breaths, postures, foods and thoughts all day long.

If the Chinese spend a lot of time practicing Tai Chi and Yogis meditate all day in yoga positions, why does the modern western woman choose this practice for only a couple of hours a week?

ChiroChi is where the Western practice of Chiropractic meets the magic of Eastern Yoga and Tai Chi. During my 32 years as a Chiropractor, I have tuned up hundreds of Yoga and Tai Chi Masters with Chiropractic Care. The valuable understanding of the position of the spinal cord and spinal nerves is very important to those who Master and teach these eastern methods of healing. Many women believe that if they spend only one hour on their spinal positions in Yoga or Tai Chi classes that they are neurologically fit. **If Yoga Masters and Tai Chi Masters go to the Chiropractor for neurological and spinal tune ups, then why don't western students of Yoga and Tai Chi understand the importance of doing the same?**

I find it difficult to understand why Western Chiropractic is so ignored when its teachings are the same as the popular eastern ones. I hear it all the time. "I don't need to go to a Chiropractor, I have no pain and I do Yoga three times a week."

Chiropractic represents the non-symptomatic approach to health and promotes holistic neurological fitness. Remember that some of your nervous system does not have pain receptors, so you can be unhealthy and not know it. Chiropractic and ChiroChi can take you from the symptomatic sickness consciousness to one of wellness. Higher levels of greatness can be achieved when you accept the lifestyle of the non-symptomatic pathway to holistic health. The ChiroChi lifestyle of greatness requires that we stay conscious of our breath, spinal positions, nutrition, thoughts and emotions all day long.

So how do we take Yoga and Tai Chi and combine them into an all-day ChiroChi lifestyle? The spinal hygiene and conscious breath work of ChiroChi is what you choose to practice when your class or DVD is over—and you choose to do it *all day long.*

Do you think that a one-hour class can heal a woman who sits at her computer in a twisted posture, clenching her jaw for six hours a day?

Do you think that a one-hour video can heal a woman who worries all day and is holding her breath while she is not practicing proper spinal hygiene?

Do you think a one-hour class three times a week or every day can undue twelve hours of negative thinking, breath holding and being hunched over a lap top or cell phone?

Do you think a one-hour-a-day-practice can undue forty eight hours of anger and resentment that some women hold onto before they allow forgiveness and gratitude to flow into their hearts?

ChiroChi is remembering to be thankful for all your lessons and gifts and to practice your spinal hygiene by tipping your chin off of your throat, stretching your shoulders backwards, relaxing your knees, balancing your hips, unclenching your jaw, taking long circular and deep spinal breaths and choosing the healthy bliss of Yoga and Tai Chi all day long. I call this reaction to life The Dancing Sacral-Cranial Spinal Breath.

You were born with a sacral-cranial pump (pelvis-head) that assists the flow of cerebral spinal fluid up and down your spinal cord from your pelvis to your head. (Refer to Autonomic Nervous System chart.) This pump is activated by our breath. When we have bad posture, and hold our breath, our sacral-cranial pump slows down and we have less energy going to our cells and more disease. Breath is life, and we need to choose to take extra breaths and hold healthy spinal postures all day long if we want to promote health in our bodies and in our lives. Here are some suggestions to help this valuable pump do its job.

The Pump

To pump the sacral-cranial breath, think of the tip of your nose and the pubic bone as moving in the same direction while you breathe.

Inhalation

When you breathe in, the tip of your nose comes up in the air and your pubic bone follows in the same direction.

Exhalation

As you breathe out, bring your nose back to neutral position and relax your pubic bone down and back.

If you are advanced in spinal fitness, you can increase these movements, but be gentle with your body. If you spend most of your day with your head down, please do not finish the breath with your head down.

The tipping of your head up, the squeezing of the shoulders backwards and the dropping of the buttocks on inhalation can be done discreetly in public. While relaxing back to a neutral position on exhalation your spine is smiling and your nervous system is happy and peaceful. You and your spine can breathe and dance all day! This can help your heart pump oxygen better, your brain to clear and increase your ability to heal.

Breath is Life, Life is Breath! We can't remove all the stress from our lives, but we can always choose to breathe into healthy spinal postures all day long. The more breaths we take, the healthier we will become. Surrender to your breath. Choose to relax and breathe!

The following breath exercises are to be done on the floor and are used by Chiropractors when they are performing Sacral-Cranial Occipital Technique. These exercises can be done at home as well.

Breath Exercise #1

POSITION 1: Lay on your back face up (supine), stretch your arms above your head. Point your toes down and take three deep, long full-body breaths.

POSITION 2: Remain face up, (as in Position 1) flex your toes toward your head, and take three deep, long, full-body breaths.

Breath Exercise #2

POSITION 1: Lie flat on your back with your arms at your sides, tilt your head back, make fists with your hands and flex your toes up toward your head. INHALE.

POSITION 2: Unclench your fists, relax your hands and point your toes downward. Return your head to the neutral position and EXHALE.

Always get up slowly from breath work to prevent dizziness.

CHOOSING THE CHIROCHI WAY OF LIFE helps women take back their power and creates a world where women are strong and healthy. Remembering to breathe while holding healing postures and having your spine dance ALL DAY LONG is a choice and you are the only one who can make these decisions.

You were born for greatness! An advanced step into greatness would be to practice honoring everything and everyone. This healing attitude stems from the consciousness that everything and everyone holds a gift and a valuable lesson. This is one way that successful healthy women choose out of the victim role and become victorious.

Relax and let go of stress! Honor yourself and live up to your highest potential.

The ChiroChi way of life is an adjunct to Chiropractic Care. When you breathe and relax into healing spinal postures, choose emotional fitness and healthy foods, you are taking out your toothbrush, brushing your spine, preventing spinal decay, and promoting wellness. Just as a dental hygienist removes plaque from your teeth, a Chiropractor removes nerve pressure during a specific adjustment. It is up to us to continue our wellness care with our teeth, nervous systems and our spines between visits and to stay conscious of its well-being. So all day long we perform the consciousness of ChiroChi and assist the Chiropractic adjustment. Many question the amount of time it takes for Chiropractic to work and for the spine to stay in place. When an orthodontist puts braces on teeth to straighten them, the prediction of time to straighten them (with steel wires) is usually about three years. Chiropractic does not have screws or steel to keep the bones in place after the Chiropractic adjustment. A ChiroChi lifestyle of holistic consciousness and spinal fitness must be adhered to if one wants to achieve a happy, high state of health.

If you are not getting fast great results you might consider having a private ChiroChi session with a ChiroChi Master. During a ChiroChi session one breathes and activates the sacral-cranial pump for over an hour. Color therapy, aromatherapy, sacral-cranial- spinal reiki and energy clearings are used to release negative memories and barriers to the nervous system's ability to create optimal health. ChiroChi Masters have the ability to read energy and can help to assist one in choosing the right diet, postures, thoughts, spinal forgiveness, and empowering questions that will increase one's ability to heal. During a ChiroChi session, a new technique called "Forgiveness Freedom Tunnels"© may be incorporated to empower the chakra energy systems and promote increased healing to the organs. ChiroChi helps people to heal on all levels.

This guidebook is dedicated to all women who want to be healthy and to all who were misguided, misinformed or chose to be powerless.

Women of all ages, your time for greatness is now and you are ready! You own the miraculous ability to heal yourself. Everything you need is inside of you. YOU are an amazing creature of love and you are only limited by your thoughts and beliefs.

The secrets to greatness have been encoded inside your nervous system. Spend time on spinal hygiene and neurological fitness and watch your body and your life change. Be the powerful woman you were created to be.

Seek out Doctors of Chiropractic and ChiroChi Masters who teach the truth about the body's natural ability to heal itself so you and your family can enjoy natural immunity and holistic neurological fitness. Practice spinal hygiene and ChiroChi all day long and enjoy a high level of feminine holistic fitness! Release toxic foods, negative thoughts and emotions that rob your power and your innate ability to heal yourself.

Thank you for reading this important information that can help women to increase their healing potential in their bodies and in their lives. Thank you in advance for passing this information on to others. Women need to re-educate themselves and express higher levels of health, wellness and greatness. Living the 8 steps in this guide book will increase women's levels of Holistic Fitness and Greatness. Educating women will create a healthier, happy world and will empower future generations.

Other Natural Holistic Healing Books by Dr. Lynn Ann Migdal

Students' Easy, Natural Guide to Greatness

A simple guide to help students increase their total fitness and health.

Wind Kissed

A self-empowering children's fantasy!

Sacred Birth Promise

An Autobiography

www.ingramcontent.com/pod-product-compliance
Lightning Source LLC
Chambersburg PA
CBHW081422270326

41931CB00015B/3374